Nadja Soares Vila Nova
Selene M. de Morais

Phytotherapeutic alternatives for the treatment of kala-azar

Nadja Soares Vila Nova
Selene M. de Morais

Phytotherapeutic alternatives for the treatment of kala-azar

Phytotherapy in the treatment of leishmaniasis: use of bioactive compounds extracted from Brazilian caatinga plants

ScienciaScripts

Imprint

Cover image: www.ingimage.com

This book is a translation from the original published under ISBN 978-613-9-69014-5.

Publisher:
Sciencia Scripts
is a trademark of
Dodo Books Indian Ocean Ltd. and OmniScriptum S.R.L publishing group

120 High Road, East Finchley, London, N2 9ED, United Kingdom
Str. Armeneasca 28/1, office 1, Chisinau MD-2012, Republic of Moldova, Europe
Printed at: see last page
ISBN: 978-620-8-24567-2

SUMMARY

1. INTRODUCTION:

Visceral leishmaniasis (VL) is an emerging and re-emerging zoonosis in tropical and subtropical regions of the world caused by the protozoan *Leishmania infantum chagasi*. In addition to humans, it affects canids, felids, rodents and marsupials and is transmitted by the phlebotomus *Lutzomia longipalpis* (ALENCAR et al., 1991).

In the New World, the main way in which the parasite is transmitted to humans and other mammalian hosts is through the bite of female dipterans of the Psychodidae family, sub-family Phlebotominae, known generically as phlebotomines. The genus *Lutzomyia* is responsible for transmitting leishmaniasis in the Americas. There are 350 cataloged species, distributed from southern Canada to northern Argentina. Of these, at least 200 occur in the Amazon basin (GILL et al., 2003). *Lutzomyia longipalpis* is the main vector of *Leishmania chagasi* in Brazil (GONTIJO; MELO, 2004).

Canine leishmaniasis is a serious problem in veterinary medicine and public health, as the dog is considered the main reservoir. The World Health Organization (WHO) indicates the euthanasia of seropositive dogs as a way of controlling leishmaniasis, however this type of approach generates discomfort with owners and discussions with animal protection organizations, and its impact on reducing cases in humans is not fully understood (NUNES et al., 2010). In Europe, four approaches are used to prevent the spread of canine leishmaniasis to other dogs and humans. The first is vaccination, the second is the use of repellents, the third is the euthanasia of seropositive animals followed by the fourth which is the treatment of these animals (AIT-OUDHIA et al., 2012).

Studies carried out using various drugs for human use have shown a remission of symptoms and a clinical cure, but they do not guarantee a parasitological cure and relapses are frequent (SOLANO-GALEGO et al., 2009). This low efficiency may be related to the animal's immune status, the pharmacokinetic properties of the drugs and the sensitivity of the different *Leishmania* strains and drug resistance (AIT-OUTHIA et al., 2012). However, the treatment of these animals is able to reduce symptoms and parasitemia, and reduce the possibility of transmission (SOLANO-GALEGO et al.,

2009).

However, in Brazil, the Ministry of Health in a Technical Note - "USE OF MEGLUMINE ANTIMONIATE IN DOGS", dated January 20, 2004, based on opinion No. 0299/2004 of the Attorney General's Office, determined that the use of medication for the treatment of leishmaniasis in dogs is prohibited when it is distributed by the Ministry of Health. An inter-ministerial ordinance, MAPA/MS 1.426/2008, bans the treatment of visceral leishmaniasis in infected or sick dogs with products for human use or products not registered with the Ministry of Agriculture, Livestock and Supply (MAPA).

2 LITERATURE REVIEW

2.1 History of Visceral Leishmaniasis

Visceral leishmaniasis (VL) was described in Greece in 1835 when it was then called "ponos" or "hapoplinakon". It was in India in 1869 that it received the name "kala-jwar" which means black fever or "kala- azar" which means black skin due to the slight increase in skin pigmentation that occurs during the disease (MARZOCHI et al., 1981).

In 1900, it was identified by Major W.B. Leishman, who described a case of a young English soldier who had returned from Dum-Dum in India, the patient showing symptoms similar to others observed by Leishman. The autopsy revealed an excessive enlargement of the spleen and histological examination revealed round or oval microorganisms with a round nucleus. These are characteristic of the amastigote forms of *Leishmania* (GILLESPIE; PEARSON, 2001).

The first case in Brazil was described by Migone in 1913. The patient was an Italian immigrant who had lived for many years in Santos, SP, and after traveling to Mato Grosso, he fell ill and was diagnosed with the disease in Paraguay (ALENCAR, 1977). It was Penna (1934) who began studying the geographical distribution of Visceral Leishmaniasis in the Americas, when he parasitologically confirmed 41 cases out of 40,000 viscerotomies examined for yellow fever from various states in Brazil.

VL in the state of Ceará had its first cases recorded by Deane and Deane (1954a) in 1934, coming from Sobral and was in the process of expanding, both in magnitude and geographically. In the 1950s, there was also a concentration of cases of allochthonous VL in the city of Sobral, where the number of diagnoses in the city exceeded the number of diagnoses in previous years in the country (DEANE; DEANE, 1954b).

Between May 1953 and August 1945, a study was carried out covering the municipalities of Sobral, Massapé, Tianguà and Viçosa do Cearà. At the time, the population of these municipalities was 1,550 and during the period studied there were 52 cases of human leishmaniasis. A study of canine leishmaniasis was also carried out in this region, where 174 dogs were examined, 7 of which tested positive. In addition to dogs, the incidence of the disease was studied in foxes in the region, identified as *Cerdocyon thous.* A total of 33 animals were examined, 10 of which came from the study site and 23 were caught in the sertao or tope de serra areas. Of the 10 foxes caught in the leishmaniasis hotspot under study, 3 were parasitized, while only 1 of the other 23 was parasitized. This indicates that there were three natural host mammals in the study area: man, the domestic dog and the fox (DEANE; DEANE, 1955).

Dogs often accompanied northeastern families on their migrations, which was proven in a survey on canine visceral leishmaniasis (CVL) in Sobral, where among the affected animals, some had been brought by their owners from rural locations, some of which were VL hotspots. This already indicated that sick men and dogs were potentially responsible for the appearance of VL in places they migrated to or passed through, as long as the transmitting phlebotoms were present in these areas (DEANE; DEANE, 1955). As in the city of Sobral, in the Jaguaribe Valley, still in the state of Ceará, some urban cases of the infection were also detected, not only in humans but also in dogs (ALENCAR et al., 1956).

2.2 Relationships between Human Visceral Leishmaniasis and Canine Visceral Leishmaniasis

The analysis of this controversial subject leads to the question of whether VL would not exist in the absence of dogs, whether eradication of the disease would be possible by controlling transmission in dogs. This aspect deserves to be analyzed, because so far in Brazil, despite the measures implemented by government agencies, epidemiological indicators show that the expected positive impact on the control of this disease has not yet been observed (FUNASA, 2002).

Nunes et al. (2001) state that although human visceral leishmaniasis (HVL) does not always follow a spatial distribution parallel to that of CVL, canine infections are more frequent than human infections and usually precede them. Most studies on HVL epidemics have found positive dogs, and there are no reports in the Brazilian literature of HVL epidemics without the presence of a positive dog (period 1953-1997) (FUNASA, 2002). Oliveira et al. (2001) found evidence that in Belo Horizonte, MG, cases of HVL occurred in places with high rates of CVL. In Belo Horizonte and Araçatuba-SP, places where HVL did not exist, it was possible to observe the introduction of the canine disease first and then the human disease (FUNASA, 2002). In Araçatuba, Assis et al. (2008) did not find a significant association between canine euthanasia and the incidence of HVL between 2000 and 2002, although the incidence of human cases tried to increase along with the rate of euthanasia in dogs. However, CVL does not seem to be the sufficient cause, but rather the necessary cause for the appearance of HVL in a region.

Rab et al. (1995) stated that in Pakistan, even with high rates of infected dogs, VLH is not related to infection in dogs, and that families with seropositive dogs have the same risk of infection as families with healthy dogs. Dietze et al. (1997) studied the impact of the removal of dogs in Espirito Santo on the transmission of VL. In this study, they chose three cities separated by a geographical barrier (mountains), all endemic for VL. In two of them, after a serological survey, all sero-reactive dogs were removed and in the control city, all the dogs were kept. Over 12 months, human seropositivity rates were measured by the Dot-Elisa test and increased from 14% to 54% in the control city and from 15% to 54% in the intervention cities. Paranhos-Silva et al. (1998), studying the effect of migration on the incidence of VL in a cohort of dogs in the state of Bahia, showed that although all seropositive dogs were eliminated from the study area, the number of reports of the disease in humans increased in the following years. These studies have shown that the criterion for eliminating dogs needs to be re-evaluated. In Barra de Guabiraba, RJ, a city endemic for VL, it has been shown that disease control measures, such as sacrificing dogs diagnosed with VL, do not influence the number of cases of the disease (CABREIRA et al., 2003).

VL in the municipality of Fortaleza has historically had a low prevalence of both canine and human leishmaniasis, but since 2001 there has been an increase in the number of VL cases, with transmission recorded in most of the city's neighborhoods (SMS, 2007).

Rondon et al. (2008) analyzed the situation of CVL between 2005 and 2007 in the different Regional Executive Secretariats (SER) into which the city of Fortaleza is divided. In this study, the author examined 1,381 animals, of which 750 were house dogs and 631 were street dogs, obtaining a seroprevalence of 21.4% (135/631) in street dogs and 26.2% (197/750) in house dogs. However, according to data provided by the Zoonosis Control Center (CCZ) in Fortaleza, between 2005 and 2007, 9002 animals were diagnosed by the CCZ and 6096 animals seropositive for leishmaniasis were euthanized.

According to the Ceará State Health Department (SESA), from 1986 to August 2012, 2006 had the highest number of human leishmaniasis cases in the state (796 cases), followed by 2007 (720 cases) (SESA, 2012). The city of Fortaleza is in an epidemiological situation of intense transmission, between 2009 and 2011 783 cases of human leishmaniasis were diagnosed with 73 deaths, and by August 2012 161 cases had already been diagnosed (SESA, 2012).

Studies in endemic areas in different regions of the country have found different rates of VL. A study carried out in Araçatuba, SP in 2005 showed that 16.7% of the 5,861 dogs euthanized that year were seropositive (ASSIS et al., 2008). In Bahia, in the municipalities of Lauro de Freitas and Camaçaria, between 2003 and 2004 there was a CVL incidence rate of 17.4% and 18.5% respectively (BARBOZA et al., 2006). Moreira et al. (2003), through a cohort study of the canine population of a neighborhood in the municipality of Jequié, BA, recorded an incidence of 11.8%. França-Silva et al. (2003), working in the municipality of Montes Claros, MG, reported an incidence of 6.4% in the canine population and Fisa et al. (1999) reported an incidence of 6.7% for canine VL in Catalonia, Spain.

Despite the fact that VL is compulsorily notifiable (i.e. mandatory), there is practically no recording of the disease by private veterinary clinics and hospitals, and the cases recorded come from animals examined by the state's CCZs. This hinders the program to combat leishmaniasis and the real knowledge of CVL in Ceará.

2.3 Medicines used to treat Visceral Leishmaniasis

The use of human medication in the treatment of dogs does not allow the parasitological cure of the animal, but it does reduce the symptoms and the amount of parasites circulating and in the skin, and contamination of phlebotomines occurs to a lesser degree (SOLANO-GALLEGO et al., 2009). Therefore, the treatment of leishmaniasis-positive animals could be considered a way of controlling visceral leishmaniasis.

For many years, emetic tartar was the only alternative for the treatment of leishmaniasis, but due to its toxic effects, difficult administration and recurrent relapses, this drug was replaced by pentavalent antimonials (MAYRINK et al., 2006). Antimonials have been used since 1945, in South America the form of antimoniate used is meglumine antimoniate (Glucantime®), and in Brazil it is used as the first-choice drug in the treatment of leishmaniasis, however liver changes and cardiac disorders are the main effects caused by the toxicity of this drug. Antimony can be detected in the hair of treated patients up to a year after the end of treatment. The use of this drug requires more than 28 days of parenteral administration and the emergence of resistance has become a serious public health problem (CROFT; COOMBS, 2003; AWASTHI et al., 2004; RATH et al., 2003; ANDERSEN et al., 2005).

This is why Tempone and Andrade (2008) developed a liposomal formulation of antimony with high efficacy and capable of reducing the total dose administered by 133 times. The routes by which antimonials enter the macrophage are still uncertain, but it is believed that the parasite's aquaglyceroporin (aquaporin 1 transporter protein) is responsible for transporting antimonials into the amastigotes (SINGH et al., 2012). Upon entering the host cell, the drug is reduced to its trivalent form (trivalent antimonial - SbIII), which induces an efflux of trypanothione and glutathione from the cells and also inhibits trypanothione reductase, causing a large loss of thiol reduction potential in the cells (BRUNTON et al., 2006). Antimony also has indirect mechanisms of action, raising cytokine levels and also DNA levels, inducing DNA damage in *vivo* (FREITAS-JUNIOR et al., 2012).

Pentamidine is a chemotherapy drug that belongs to the diamide group and is used as an alternative in cases where the individual does not respond to treatment with antimoniate. However, its nephrotoxicity and cadiotoxicity also limit the use of this drug, and the patient may die. There are two pentamidine salts, pentamidine isethionate (Pentamidine®), available in the Americas and Europe, and pentamidine mesylate (Lomidine®). Their mechanism of action has not been fully elucidated (RATH et al., 2003; PAULA et al., 2003; BLUM et al., 2004). Andersen et al. (2005) compared treatments with antimoniate and pentamidine and observed that under identical conditions, pentamidine was less effective than glucantime.

Amphoterine B is an antifungal antibiotic derived from *Streptomyces nodosus* and used to treat systemic fungal infections. This drug is used to treat leishmaniasis in cases of resistance to first-choice drugs. This drug is able to bind to the ergosterol present in the *Leishmania* membrane, resulting in an increase in the parasite's cell permeability and the consequent loss of small chaperones such as K^+ (ORDONEZ- GUTIÉRREZ et al., 2007; RATH et al., 2003). However, amphotericin B has a low gastrointestinal absorption capacity and hydrophobic characteristics, and can also interact with mammalian cell pathways causing dysfunction (ROY et al., 2012), with its main side effect being nephrotoxicity (MOTTA; SAMPAIO, 2012).

One way of trying to reduce toxicity and resistance to leishmanicidal drugs is to develop new formulations with the aim of targeting the drug to the macrophage. Liposomes have been used in conjunction with amphotericin B. Liposomes are drug carrier systems that are capable of delivering high doses of the drug to the target cell (TEMPONE; ANDRADE, 2008). Liposomal amphotericin B reduces side effects and has excellent therapeutic efficacy rates even in individuals who have not responded to treatment with antimonials (PAULA et al., 2003; MOTTA; SAMPAIO, 2012). However, the high cost of this drug limits its use in underdeveloped and developing countries (ORDONES-GUTIÉRREZ et al., 2007). In developed countries, liposomal amphotericin B is used as the drug of first choice and is also the only drug approved by the American Food and Drug Administration (FDA) (VAN GRIENSVEN; DIRO, 2012).

A major advance in the treatment of leishmaniasis was the development of miltefosine, which was approved in 2002 as the first leishmanicidal drug to be used orally (DORLO et al., 2012; PALADIN LABS INC., 2010). Mylefosine, an alkylphospholipid, was originally developed as a drug for the treatment of cancer (CROFT; COOMBS, 2003) and its action against leishmaniasis was quickly recognized. Its toxicity is not that high, however it is extremely teratogenic and in women treatment is carried out in non-pregnant women who agree to take contraceptives during, and three months after the end of treatment (SOTO et al., 2004; SUNDAR et al., 2012), other side effects are gastrointestinal dysfunction, headaches and increased liver enzymes (BLUM et al., 2004). Its mechanism of action acts on lipid metabolism causing apoptosis of the parasite, it also acts directly on the host cell stimulating the production of nitric oxide synthase 2 (iNOS2) which catalyzes the production of nitric oxide (NO) and kills the parasite inside the macrophage (FREITAS-JUNIOR et al., 2012).

Paromomycin is an aminoglycoside antibiotic that was rediscovered as a leishmanicidal agent in the 1980s and has been used successfully parenterally and topically (RATH et al., 2003; DORLO et al., 2012). Its mechanism of action has not yet been fully elucidated, however it is believed that paromomycin binds to the glycans of leishmania, suggesting that mitochondria are a primary target (SINGH et al., 2012).

Aloupurinol is an analog of hypoxanthine and is normally used in association with antimony (BLUM et al., 2004). This drug has low toxicity but is ineffective in controlling the infection (RATH et al., 2003). This drug is used as a substrate by various enzymes in the purine pathway in trypanosomids, being incorporated into the intermediate nucleotides and nucleic acids of the parasite (CROFT; COOMBS, 2003).

2.4 Use of natural products as alternatives for the treatment of Leishmaniasis

Drug development follows three lines, the first explores the parasite's metabolic pathways to find targets and develop synthetic compounds, the second is the study of other drugs already on the market with unknown leishmanicidal activity (e.g. cancer drugs) and the third is focused on the use of medicinal plants as a source of anti-protozoan molecules (LINDOSO et al., 2012).

2.4.1 Medicinal plants

Plants are important sources of drug discovery, especially with regard to anti-parasitic drugs, due to the association between the coexistence of parasites, living beings and medicinal plants (ANTHONY et al., 2005). Natural products offer molecules with a profound impact on human health, and nature produces infinite secondary metabolites with distinct biological properties. Several studies have already validated the effect of natural products as rich potential sources of new and selective agents for the treatment of tropical diseases caused by protozoa and other parasites (MISHRA et al., 2009).

Observation of the therapeutic properties of plants has led to research into the active principles of various plant species. The exploration of plant resources can lead to the identification of valuable secondary metabolites that can serve as drugs or lead to the development of new therapeutic substances (GOBBO-NETO; LOPES, 2007). Plant metabolism is made up of a set of chemical reactions that are continuously taking place in cells. The synthesis of compounds such as amino acids, sugars, fatty acids and nucleotides, which are essential for plant survival, is part of primary metabolism. On the other hand, compounds synthesized by other routes, which appear to have no direct relationship with plant survival, are part of secondary metabolism (MORAIS; BRAZ-FILHO, 2007). It is now known that many of the substances produced by secondary metabolism have important biological properties and are directly involved in the mechanisms that allow the plant to adapt to its environment. Many secondary metabolites have various biological functions, such as defense against herbivores and microorganisms, protection against UV rays, attraction of pollinators or seed-dispersing animals (FUMAGALI et al., 2008).

Due to the limited viability of effective leishmanicidal chemotherapy drugs in endemic areas, a large part of the population living in these places relies on medicinal plants which are used in popular treatments to treat and alleviate the symptoms of leishmaniasis (CHAN-BACAB; PENA-RODRIGUEZ, 2001). These plants have secondary metabolites that can act on and destroy invading agents, but these substances are often unknown and may offer alternative treatments for leishmaniasis.

Secondary metabolites such as alkaloids, terpenoids and flavonoids, once considered inactive, are now important tools in the treatment of protozoa. Compounds that stimulate the immune system are useful when used as adjuvants in the treatment of certain diseases caused by fungi, bacteria and protozoa, such as leishmaniasis. In the latter case, chemical and immunopharmacological studies have been carried out with the aim of finding new compounds that are less toxic, more economically viable, have a specific effect and reverse the parasite's resistance to drugs (BERGMANN et al., 1997).

Brazil is the country with the greatest plant genetic diversity in the world, with more than 55,000 cataloged species (AZEVEDO; SILVA, 2006). According to Simoes et al. (2004), only 8% of this biological percentage has been studied for bioactive compounds and 1,100 plant species have been evaluated for their medicinal properties. Of these, 590 plants have been registered with the Ministry of Health for commercialization.

However, it is only in the last 30 years that the efficacy and mechanism of action of drugs derived from plants have been seriously studied (ANTHONY et al., 2005). Some authors have been researching new alternatives for the treatment of leishmaniasis in nature, which is a great source of drugs used in the treatment of various diseases. Based on popular use, these authors are looking for drugs with lower toxicity and cost extracted from plants and microorganisms.

However, there are several aspects that limit research into natural products: (1) low viability of compounds, in general the substances extracted from plants are low in quantity and difficult to extract; (2) high structural complexity, various stereoisomers; (3) lack of continuity in research, most research is not part of programs to develop new drugs, there is a lack of continuity in research; (4) isolated compounds often do not show activity and require monitoring to improve these activities (MISHRA et al... 2009), 2009).

As part of the search for new and better drugs with high viability and low toxicity, the Tropical Diseases Program of the World Health Organization (WHO) has considered research into the use of plants in the treatment of leishmaniasis to be essential and a high priority (WHO, 2012).

2.4.2 Annonaceae

Annona muricata (Figure 1) is a plant commonly found in Brazil and traditionally used to treat cancer. It belongs to the *Annonaceae* family and is popularly known as Graviola (GEORGE et al., 2012; HAMIZAH et al., 2012). It is used to combat worms, fever, diarrhea and dysentery, as well as having antioxidant properties (BASKAR et al., 2007). The leaves have antispasmodic, hypotensive, antiparasitic, antidiarrheal and rheumatological properties (ARTHUR et al., 2012; SOUSA et al., 2010). The infusion of the leaves also has antiplasmodic, astringent and gastric, renal and hepatoprotective properties, in addition to its action against jaundice (ARTHUR et al., 2012).

The leaves of *A. muricata* have been the subject of several studies indicating various secondary metabolites belonging to the acetogenin class (YUAN et al., 2003). The high potential, selectivity, chemical variety, biological diversity and action of this class of compounds against antibiotic-resistant agents could make these substances important in the fight against parasitic agents.

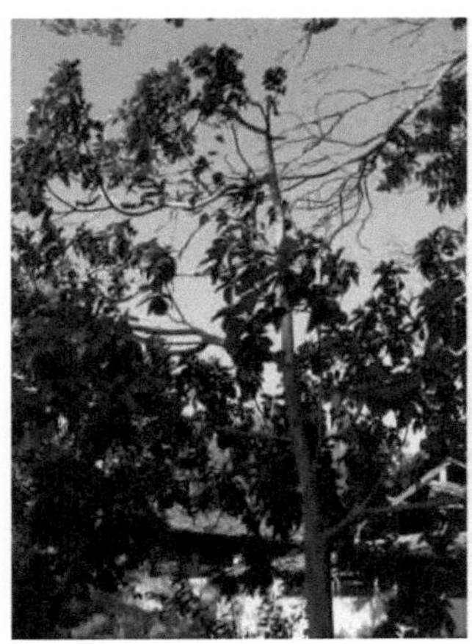
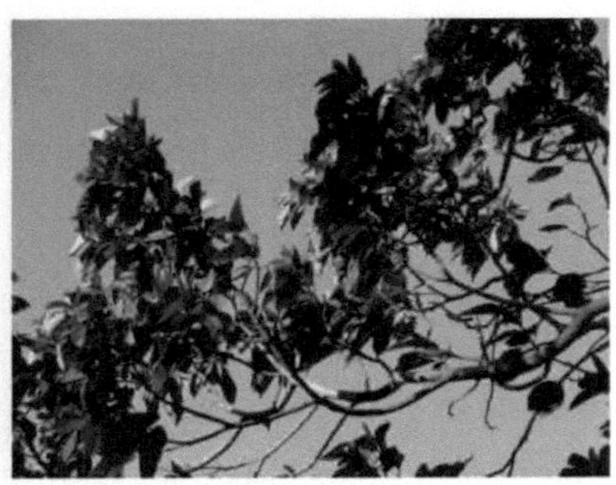

Figure 1. The *Annona muricata* plant. Source: Vila-Nova, 2012

Annona squamosa (Figure 2) is popularly called ata, pinha, fruta do conde and its pharmacological preparations are known worldwide. It is an excellent source of calcium and has insecticidal properties. The leaves are used as a purgative and their decoction is used to treat diabetes and relieve rheumatic pain (PATEL et al., 2012).

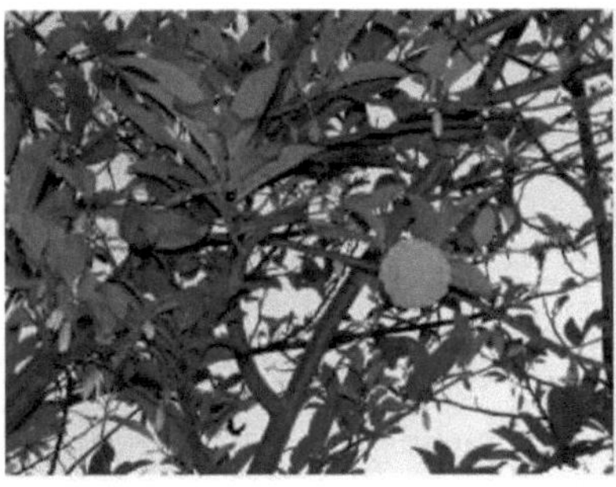 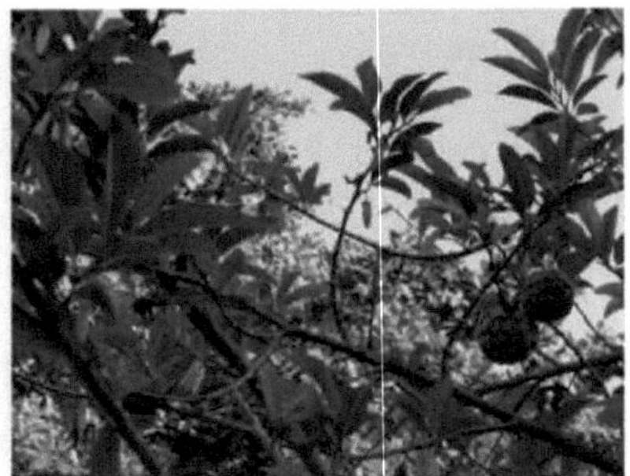

Figure 2. The *Annona squamosa* plant. Source: Vila-Nova, 2012

This plant is known for the potent secondary metabolites found in all its parts. One of its best-known properties is anti-cancer (SRIVASTAVA et al., 2011). Its seeds, which are often thrown away, have anti-ovulatory and abortifacient (PANDLEY; BARVE, 2011), anthelmintic (SOUZA et al., 2007); the ethanolic extract has insecticidal (KUMAR et al., 2010), hypoglycemic (MUJEEB et al., 2009), molucid (MRITA et al., 2001), antibacterial (PATEL et al., 2012); the aqueous extract has antioxidant (KALEEM et al., 2006), anti-inflammatory (CHAVAN et al., 2010) activity, these are just a few examples of the many applications of *A. squamosa*.

This plant belongs to the *Annonaceae* family and produces various secondary metabolites, including alkaloids and acetogenins, which are responsible for the plant's various activities.

2.4.2.1 Acetogenins

Acetogenins, widely found in Annonaceae, are responsible for most of the pharmacological activities attributed to these plants (UPADHYAY; AHMAD, 2012). One of the most studied activities of acetogenins is their anti-cancer activity. Alvarez-Gonzalez et al. (2008) induced the formation of crypts in the colon of mice and observed that acetogenins were able to reduce these crypts; another study concluded that acetogenins cause depletion of ATP production by pancreatic carcinogenic cells (TORRES et al., 2012); in a third study Atawodi et al. (2011) proved the action of acetogenins on prostate cancer cells.

Other actions can also be associated with the presence of these secondary metabolites present in extracts made from different parts of Annonaceae. Among the most diverse activities, we can mention the action against herpes simplex (PADMA et al., 1998), hypotensive (NWOKOCHA et al., 2012), larvicidal against *Aedes aegypti* larvae and molucicidal against *Biomphalaria glabrata*, the intermediate host of *Schistosoma mansoni* (GRZYBOWSKI et al., 2012; LUNA et al., 2005), *antiplasmodium* against *Plasmodium falciparum* (BOYOM et al., 2011) and antimicrobial (LIMA et al., 2006). The acetogenins of the Anonaceae have demonstrated a great leishmanicidal effect against various species of *Leishmania*, and stand out in quantity and variety.

From the roots of *A. muricata*, cis-solamine A was isolated, an acetogenin with a mono-tetrahydrofuran ring and which showed mitochondrial complex I inhibitory activity (KONNO et al., 2008); also isolated from the roots were cohibins A and B, and sabadelin, all with antipasitory action and mitochondrial complex I inhibitors (GLEYE et al., 1997; GLEYE et al., 1998). Yu et al. (1998) isolated annonacin *A* and annonacin from the seeds of *A. muricata*, and Jaramillo et al. (2000) isolated these same acetogenins from the extract of the pericarp of this same plant, and confirmed their leishmanicidal activity against *L. panamensis* and *L. braziliensis*; another study isolated annonacin from the seeds of this plant and identified its leishmanicidal activity against *L. panamensis* (ARANGO et al., 2000). From the leaves of this species, Kim et al. (1998) isolated and identified two acetogenins with a mono-tetrahydrofuran ring, muricoreacin and murihexocin. Calderon et al. (2010) using a crude extract of this plant found leishmanicidal activity against amastigote forms of *L. mexicana.*

A trihydroxylated acetogenin with two tetrahydrofuranic rings and an α,β-unsaturated lactonic ring with 37 carbon atoms was isolated from the seeds of *A. squamosa* (Figure 3), which has antihelminthic properties against *Haemonchus contortus*, the main nematode of sheep and goats in northeastern Brazil (SOUZA et al., 2008). This substance has shown anti-helminthic action against promastigote and amastigote forms of *L. chagasi* (VILA-NOVA et al., 2011).

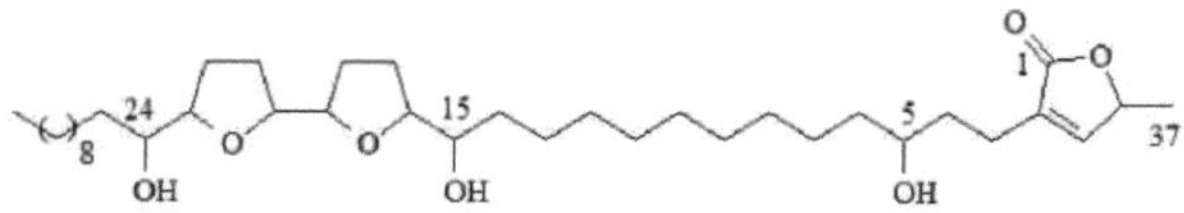

Figure 3. Trihydroxylated acetogenin with two tetrahydrofuranic rings and α,β-unsaturated lactonic ring of 37 carbon atoms isolated from *A. squamosa* seeds.

The mechanism of action of acetogenins has not been fully elucidated. Acetogenins, which are potent inhibitors of mitochondrial complex I, inhibit NADH ubiquinone oxidoreductase, an essential enzyme in complex I. This inhibition induces oxidative phosphorylation in the mitochondria of the cell (BERMEJO et al., 2005; GRANDIC et al., 2004). Studies in the literature have shown that these substances act directly on the ubiquinone catalytic site within complex I and on microbial glucose dehydrogenase. They also inhibit the NADH oxidase linked to ubiquinone, peculiar to the plasma membranes of cancer cells (BERMEJO et al., 2005). Even though the mitochondrial complex has not been characterized in *Leishmania*, studies suggest that mitochondrial complexes I, II, III and IV are present in the electron transfer pathway and that oxidative phosphorylation is processed with high bioenergetic efficiency (GRANDIC et al., 2004).

2.4.2.2 Alkaloids

Alkaloids are complex organic nitrogen compounds derived from amino acids that undergo decarboxylation and usually have a variety of biological actions. The main amino acid precursors of alkaloids are L-lysine, L-ornithine, L-tyrosine, L-tryptophan, L-histidine, L-phenylalanine as well as nicotinic acid and anthranilic acid (ANISZEWSKI, 2007). Building blocks of the acetate and shikimate pathways are also incorporated into the structure of alkaloids. There are also a large number of alkaloids that acquire their nitrogen via the transamination reaction, incorporating only the nitrogen atom of the amino acid. The term pseudo-alkaloid is often used to distinguish this group (DEWICK, 2002). The common alkaloids in Annonaceae are of the isoquinolinic and benzylisoquinolinic types, which are biosynthetically derived from tyrosine.

Alkaloids are the class of metabolites with the highest number of compounds with leishmanicidal activity, and also comprise the largest class of secondary metabolites from plants. These metabolites play an important role in the defense against various microorganisms, possessing a remarkable variety of pharmacological activities (Calderon et al, 2009). Among the activities of the alkaloids are anti-tuberculosis (KISHORE et al., 2009), anti-cancer (MIN et al., 2010), against larval stages of nematodes (SATOU et al., 2002), molucidal (BAGALWA et al., 2010) and anti-bacterial (MANEERAT et al., 2012). Recent studies point to these products as potential sources of drugs against leishmaniasis. Several alkaloids are reported to have excellent leishmanicidal activities, however none of them have been evaluated in clinical studies or are designed for future clinical application (MISHRA et al., 2009).

Bhakuni et al. (1972) isolated the alkaloid anonaine from the bark and seeds of *A. squamosa* (Figure 4), in which Queiroz et al. (1996) demonstrated leishmanicidal activity against *L. donovani and L. amazonenses*. Bhakuni et al. (1979) isolated xylopine and O-methylarmeparvine alkaloids from the leaves of the same plant (Figure 4). The leishmanicidal action of xylopin against *L. mexicana* and *L. pananmensis* was described by Montenegro et al. (2003); the leishmanicidal action of O-methylarmeparvine against *L. chagasi* was described by Vila-Nova et al. (2011).

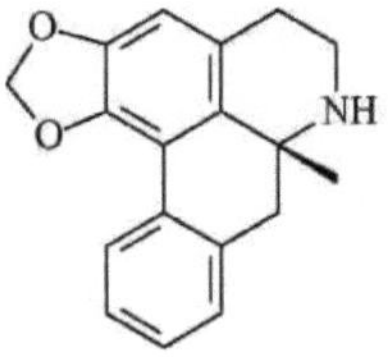

I

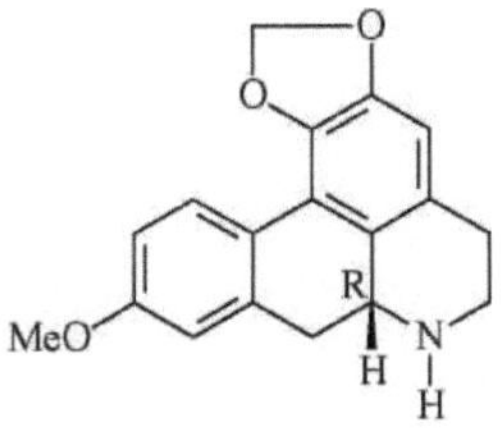

II

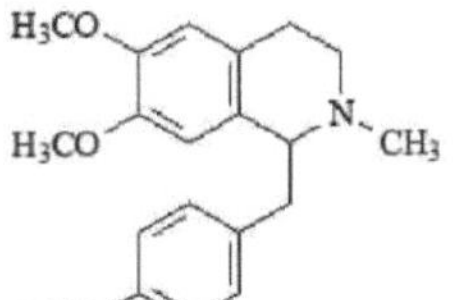

III

Figure 4: Chemical structure of (I) Anonaine, (II) Xylopine and (III) O-methylarmeparvine.

The mechanism of action of alkaloids is not fully understood, but Fournet et al. (2000) observed that bisbenzylisoquinolinic alkaloids inhibit an essential antioxidant enzyme in *Leishmania*, trypanothione reductase. Chan-Bacan and Pena-Rodriguez (2001) propose that the mechanism of action of indole alkaloids is by inhibiting the parasite's respiratory chain, and Mishra et al. (2009) propose that, because the structure of naphthylisoquinoline alkaloids is similar to miltefosine, death by apoptosis would be a possible mechanism of action.

2.4.3 - Dimorphandra gardneriana

D. gardneriana, popularly known as faveira or fava D'anta (Figure 5), is a typical plant of the Brazilian cerrado and caatinga, and is found in Ceará and the Chapada do Araripe (PIRES et al., 2010). This species is a major producer of rutin, a flavonoid with various pharmacological activities and is widely exported by Brazil (CUNHA et al., 2009).

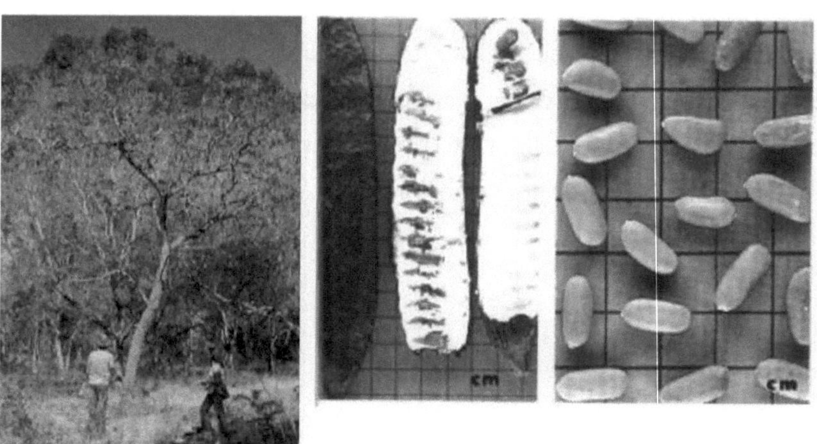

Figure 5: The plant and seeds of *Dimorphandragardneriana*. Source: icaro, 2003

2.4.3.1 - Quercetin

Quercetin (Figure 6) is an outstanding member of the flavonoid group and, due to its antioxidant action, its therapeutic performance has been mentioned by several authors in the fight against oxidative stress. Its pharmacological effect is due to its action in inhibiting certain enzymes and its antioxidant capacity (MILTERSTEINER et al.,

2003), it also acts by interacting with DNA topoisomerases (SEN et al., 2006). Its various pharmacological activities include anti-cancer and sensitization of cancer cells resistant to traditional treatments (BORSKA et al., 2012); anti-inflammatory (LIN et al., 2012) and anti-viral (SAVOV et al., 2006). *In vitro* studies have shown that quercetin and other flavonoids strongly inhibit the production of Nitric Oxide and Tumor Necrosis Factor by Kupffer cells when stimulated by injury. Flavonoids, by directly combating active oxygen species or increasing the liver's capacity to react to them, could contribute to reducing hepatic oxidative damage and the formation of fibrosis caused by biliary obstruction (MILTERSTEINER et al, 2003).

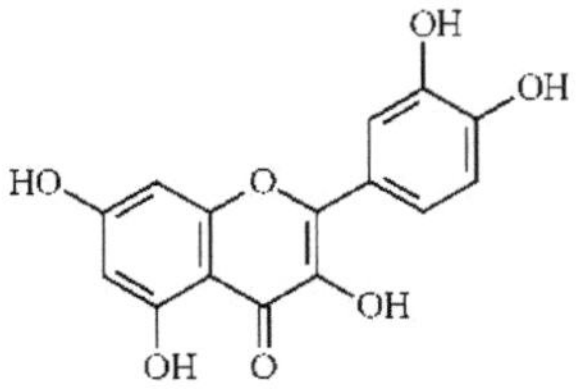

Figure 6: Representation of the molecular structure of quercetin.

Quercetin can be found in a number of plants, but the study of the leishmanicidal activity of this isolated flavonoid is still lacking. Muzitano et al. (2006) observed that quercetin isolated from *Kalanchoe pinnata, a* plant commonly known as saiào, exhibited leishmanicidal activity.

Ieishmanicidal against *L. amazonenses. The* inhibition of arginase by quercetin may be an important mechanism of action against various species of *Leishmania*, since arginase synthesizes arginine into ornithine and urea, where ornithine is essential for cell proliferation (SILVA et al., 2012).

2.4.3.2 - Rutin

Rutin (Figure 7) is a glycosidic flavonoid belonging to an important class of flavonoids found widely in nature. It is therapeutically important because it normalizes the resistance and permeability of capillary vessel walls and inhibits the formation of free radicals at various stages (PATHAK et al., 1991).

Among the therapeutic importance of rutin are: anti-allergic (SHEN et al., 2012); procarcinogenic, reducing the induction of DNA damage in liver cells (MARCARINI et al., 2011); antioxidant (KIM et al., 2011) and anti-inflammatory (SELLOUM et al., 2003).

This flavonoid inhibits the process of free radical formation in various stages, by reacting with superoxide ion and lipid peroxyl radicals, and by forming a complex with iron which catalyzes the formation of active oxygen radicals (PATHAK et al., 1991), and is non-toxic (AFANASE'EV et al., 1989). The anti-inflammatory action of this flavonoid is due to its ability to inhibit enzymes involved in the inflammatory signaling process, such as cyclooxygenase and lipoxygenase (SELLOUM et al., 2003).

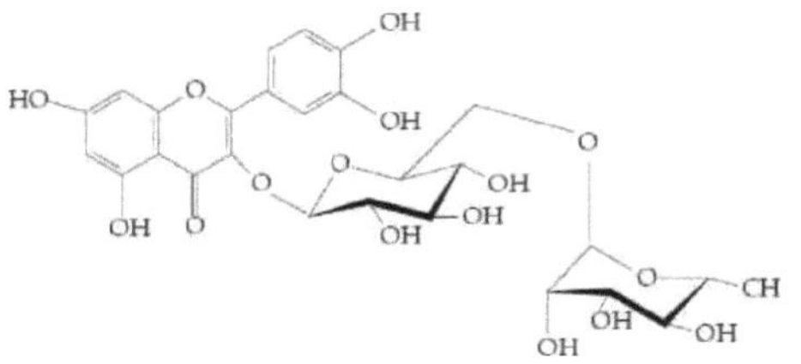

Figure 7. Representation of the molecular structure of Rutin.

Studies in the search for new vaccines against visceral leishmaniasis have used rutin as an adjuvant in their composition with promising results (OLIVEIRA-FREITAS et al., 2006).

2.4.4 - Platymiscium floribundum

P. floribundum is a common plant in northeastern Brazil and is popularly known as sacambu or jacarandà do litoral (Figure 8). This species is used by the population as an anti-inflammatory and its wood has commercial value in the furniture industry (FALCÂO et al., 2005).

The phytochemical importance of this plant includes the presence of isoflavonoids with pharmacological potential and antiviral, antifungal and anticancer biological activities (MILITÂO et al., 2006; FALCÂO et al., 2005; VALLILO et al., 2007).

The chemical study of this species revealed the presence of flavonoids, isoflavonoids and coumarins as the main constituents, the second largest class of compounds being coumarins, with a total of ten compounds identified (FALCÂO, 2003).

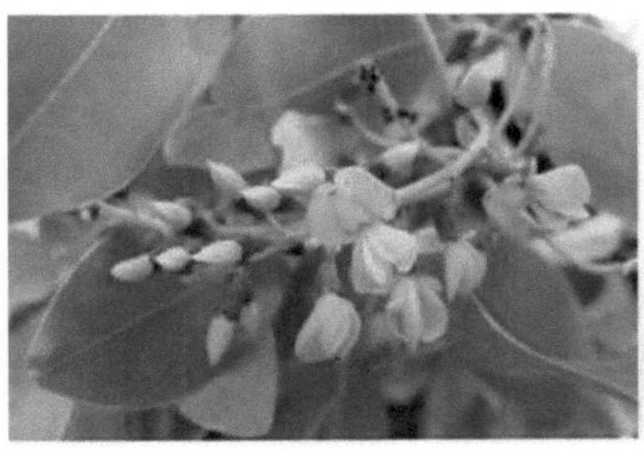 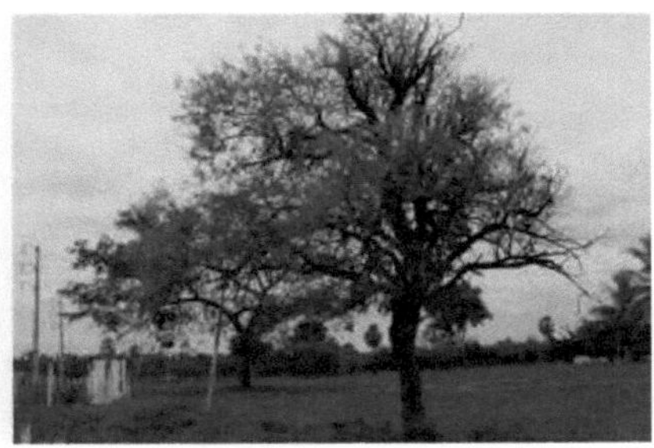

Figure 8. The flowers of the *Platymisciym floribundum* plant. Source: Falcao, 2003

2.4.4.1 Coumarins

Coumarins are part of a group of natural phenols found in various vegetables such as citrus fruits, tomatoes, legumes and green tea (BILGIN et al., 2011). Hundreds of coumarins have been isolated from plants and some of them are synthesized in the laboratory (HOULT; PAYA, 1996; MANHAS et al., 2006). This class of phenols has a variety of functions with therapeutic potential for various diseases (KONTOGIORGIS et al., 2012), including anti-cancer (KIM et al., 2012), hepatoprotective (BILGIN et al., 2011), anti-HIV (HUANG et al., 2005), antibacterial (JAISWAL et al., 2012) and hypotensive (GILANI et al., 2000) activities.

Several coumarins show leishmanicidal activity, Iranshahi et al. (2007) isolated two sesquiterpene coumarins and proved their activity against *L. major*, also with activity against this same species of *Leishmania*, auraptene (Figure 9) isolated from *Esenbeckia febrifuga* (NAPOLITANO et al., 2004), Ahua et al. (2004) isolated eight furanocoumarins and one coumarin from the roots of *Thamnosma rhodesicca* and demonstrated their activity against *L. major*, and *in vivo* leshmanicidal activity was demonstrated by Tiuman et al. (2012) who analyzed the action of the coumarin mammea A/BB in oral and topical treatments in mice.

BALB/c infected with *L. amazonenses*, data similar to that of Ferreira et al. (2010) who isolated and confirmed the activity of two coumarins from the bark of *Helietta apicupata* against this same species of *Leishmania*.

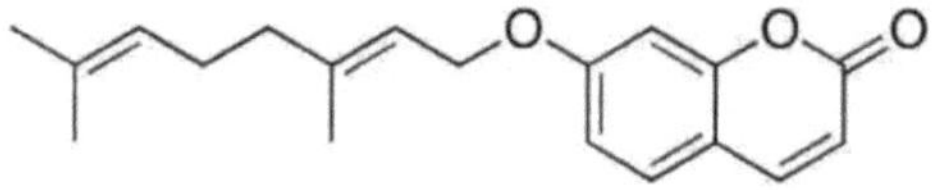

Figure 9. Chemical structure of auraptene.

Scoparone (6,7-dimethoxycoumarin) (Figure 10) is a coumarin with anti-allergic (CHOI; YAN, 2009), dopamine release inducing (YANG et al., 2010), gastric mucosa protective (CHOI et al., 2012), anti-asthmatic (FANG et al., 2003) activity, however there is a lack of research into the leishmanicidal activity of this coumarin.

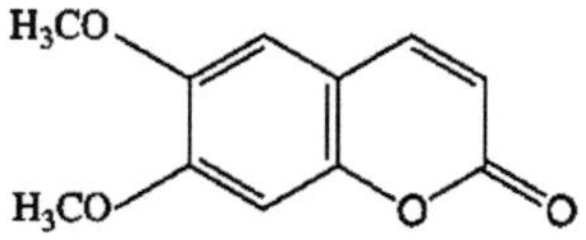

Figure 10. Chemical structure of scoparone.

2.4.5 - Components of essential oils - Monoterpenoids and phenylpropanoids

2.4.5.1 - Eugenol

Eugenol (Figure 11) is a pharmacologically very active methoxylated phenylpropanoid phenol, abundantly found in the essential oil of *Eugenia caryophyllus* (clove) (JIROVETZ et al., 2006), in essential oils of some plants from the Brazilian Northeast such as *Dicipelium cariophyllatum* (the Maranhao carnation or cravinho),

Croton zenhtneri (cinnamon wedge) and *Ocimum gratissimum* (lavender) (CRAVEIRO et al., 1981; UEDA-NAKAMURA et al., 2006).

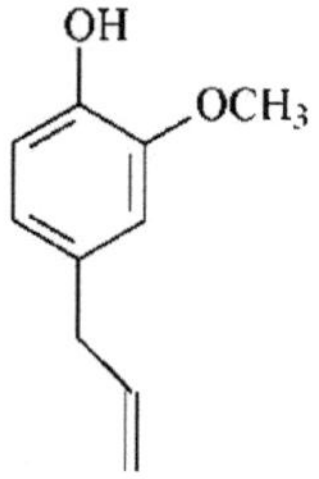

Figura 11. Representation of the molecular structure of Eugenol.

Due to its complex molecular structure, eugenol has several proven pharmacological actions such as antifungal (NAIR et al., 2012); anthelmintic (PESSOA et al., 2002); insecticidal (MACIEL et al., 2010); it is also used in dental practices as a topical antiseptic, analgesic, and to confer pharmacological properties to root canal fillings, as it has a bactericidal action and is therefore effective in the treatment of some infectious diseases in the oral cavity (MARKOWITZ et al., 1992; ESCOBAR, 2002). The eugenol-rich essential oil of *Ocimum gratissimum* showed leishmanicidal activity against *L. amazonenses,* causing mitochondrial alterations such as swelling, disorganization of the inner membrane and an increase in the number of crystals (UEDA-NAKAMURA et al., 2006), as well as pure eugenol, which also has leishmanicidal action (ARANGO et al., 2012).

Eugenol has an inhibitory activity on cyclooxygenases and prostaglandins, enzymes involved in inflammatory and carcinogenic processes, and also has the ability to induce cell lysis due to the increased loss of proteins and lipids caused by damage to the cell membrane (KAMATOU et al., 2012).

2.4.5.2 - Thymol

Thymol (figure 12) is a monoterpenoid phenol found in various plants such as *Thymus eriocalyx* and *Thymus x-porlock*. In northeastern Brazil, it is found mainly in the essential oil of *Lippia sidoides*. It is irritating to the gastric mucosa and fat or alcohol increase its absorption (BOTELHO et al., 2007).

Its therapeutic activities include antimicrobial (GUARDA et al., 2011), anti-inflammatory and healing (RIELLA et al., 2012), fungicidal (AHMAD et al., 2010), antioxidant (UNDERGER et al., 2009) and has a negative inotropic action due to the reduction of calcium in the sarcoplasm of the reticulum due to its combination of inducing calcium release and inhibiting the calcium pump (SZENTANDRÂSSY et al., 2004).

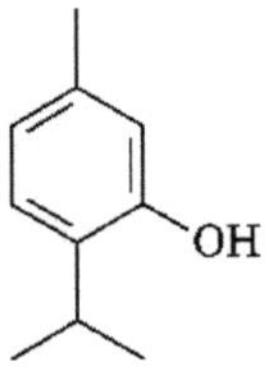

OH

Figura 12. Representation of the molecular structure of thymol.

Robledo et al. (2005) validated the *in vitro* and *in vivo* leishmanicidal activity of thymol and its structural derivatives against *Leishmania panamensis*. In another study, Medeiros et al. (2011) observed the inhibitory action of *Lippia sidoides* oil against *L. amazonenses*.

2.4.5.3 Synthetic Derivatives of Eugenol and Thymol

Thymol is a derivative of p-cymene and several derivatives have leishmanicidal activity. In the study carried out by Robledo et al.

(2005), thymol had its structure chemically modified and its derivatives were evaluated against the promastigote and amastigote forms of *L. panamensis*, proving the inhibitory activity of thymol derivatives. Eugenol is a phenylproponoid whose leishmanicidal activity has been extensively studied. Arango et al. (2012) synthesized and evaluated the action against *L. panamensis* of six eugenol hybrids, finding better inhibitory activity than eugenol in three of the six hybrids studied.

Thus, it is assumed that derivatives of thymol and eugenol may have better leishmanicidal activity than the pure substance, so obtaining derivatives by the benzoylation (Fig. 13) and acetylation (Fig. 14) processes may enable better chemotherapeutic activities and lower toxicity.

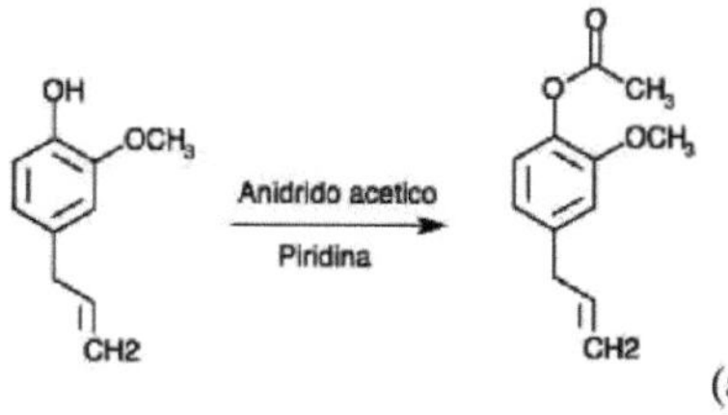

OH
OCH_3
Anidrido acetico
Piridina
CH2
O
CH_3
OCH_3
CH2
(a)

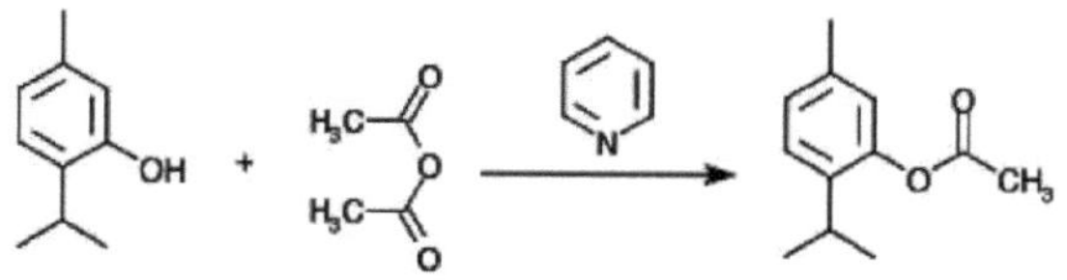

OH
+
H_3C
O
O
H_3C
O
N
O
O
CH_3
(b)

Figure 13. Processes of (a) Eugenol Acetylation and (b) Thymol Acetylation

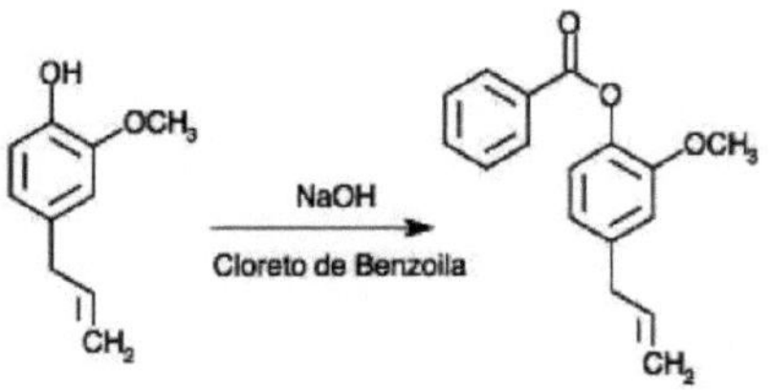

(a)

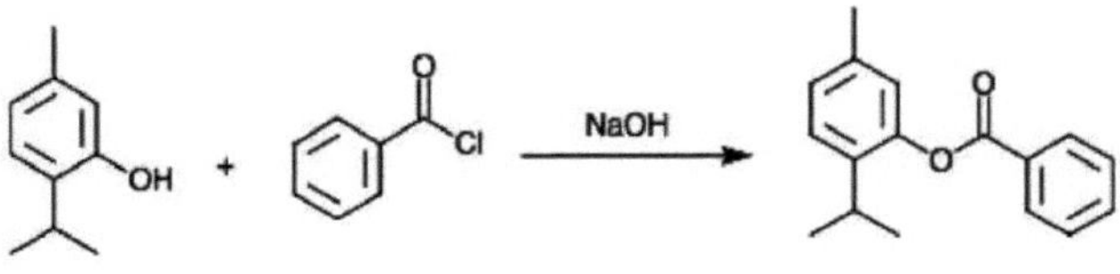

(b)

Figure 14. Processes of (a) Eugenol benzoylation and (b) Thymol benzoylation.

BIBLIOGRAPHICAL REFERENCES:

[SESA] Ceará State Health Department. Epidemiological Bulletin, Visceral Leishmaniasis, 2012.

[SMS]. Secretaria Municipal de Saùde: Relatório de gestao de 2006 da Secretaria Municipal de Saùde de Fortaleza - Health, quality of life and the ethics of care. 2007.

AFANAS'EV, I.B., DOROZHIKO, A.I., BRODSKI, A.V., KOSTYUK, V.A., POTAPOVITCH, A.I. Chelating and free radical scavenging mechanisms of nhibitory action of rutin and quercetin in lipid peroxidation. Biochem Pharmacol, v. 38, n. 11, p. 1763-1769, 1989.

Ait-Oudhia, K., Gazanion, E., Sereno, D., Oury, B., Depet, J.P., Pratlong, F. *In vitro* susceptibility to antimonials and amphotericin B of *Leishmania infantum* strains isolated from dogs in a region lacking drug selection pressure. Veterinary Parasitology 187:386-393, 2012.

ALALI, F.Q., LIU; X.X., MCLAUGHLIN; E J.L. Annonaceous acetogenins: recent progress. J Nat Prod., v. 62, n. 3, p. 504-540, 1999

ALENCAR, J. E., Calazar Canino: contribuiçao para o estudo da epidemiologia do calazar no Brasil, Fortaleza: {s. n.}, 1959.

ALENCAR, J. E.; DIETZE, R. Visceral leishmaniasis. In: VERONESI, R. Doenças Infecciosas e Parasitàrias. 8 ed. Rio de Janeiro: Guanabara Koogan. 706-717, 1991.

ALENCAR, J. E.; HOLANDA, D.; CAVALCANTE, J. D. N. Visceral leishmaniasis in the Jaguaribe Valley, Cearà. Revista Brasileira Malariologia e Doenças Tropicais, v.8, p.33-48, 1956.

ALENCAR, J.E. Visceral Leishmaniasis in Brazil. Rev. de. Med. da Universidade Federal do Cearà. v.17, p.129-148, 1977.

ALVAREZ-GONZALEZ, I., GARCiA-AGUIRRE, K.K, MARTINO-ROARO, M., ZEPEDA-VALLEJO, G., MADRIGAL-BUJAIDAR, E. Anticarcinogenic and genotoxic effects produced by acetogenins isolated from *Annona muricata*. Toxicology Letters, v. 118, p. S228, 2008

Alvarez-Gonzalez, I., Garcia-Aguirre, K.K., Martino-Roaro, L., Zepeda-Vallejo, G., Madrigal-Bujaidar, E. Anticarcinogenic and genotoxic effects produced by acetogenins isolated from *Annona muricata*. Toxicology letters 180:32-46, 2008.

ALVES, W.A; BEVILACQUA, P. D. Quality of diagnosis of canine visceral leishmaniasis in epidemiological surveys: an epidemic in Belo Horizonte, Minas Gerais, Brazil, 1993-1997. Cad. Saùde Pùblica, v. 20, n. 1, p. 259-265, 2004

Andersen, E.M., Cruz-Saldarriaga, M., LLanos-Cuentas, A., Luz-Cjuno, M., Echevarria, J., Miranda-Verastegui, C., Colina, O., Berman, J.D. Comparison of meglumine antimoniate and pentamidine for peruvian cutaneous leishmaniasis. Am. J. Trp. Med. Hyg. 72(2):133-137, 2005

ANISZEWSKI, T. Alkaloids - Secrets of Life. 1ed p. 334, 2007

Anthony, J., Fyfe, L., Smith, H. Plant active components - a resource for antiparasitic agents? Trends in Parasitology 21: 462-468, 2005.

Arango, G.J., Dickson, J.S., Vélez, I.D., Munoz, D.L. Actividad leishmanicida de Annonacina, aislada *de Annona muricata* contra *Leishmania panamensis*. Vitae 7:3842, 2000.

Arthur, F.K.N., Woode, E., Terlabi, E.O., Larbie, C. Evaluation of hepatoprotective effect of aqueous extract of *Annona muricata* (Linn.) leaf against carbon tetrachloride and acetaminophen-induced liver damage. Journal of Natural Pharmaceuticals 3:25-30, 2012.

ASSIS, F. D.; PIRES, M. M.; SILVA, K. M.; GONÇALVES FILHO, J.; PERRI, S. H. V.; NUNES, C. M. Relationship between dog euthanasia and the incidence of human visceral leishmaniasis in an endemic area. Veterinària e Zootecnia, v.15, p.85, 2008.

Atawodi, S.E. Nigerian foodstuffs with prostate cancer chemopreventive polyphenols. Infectious agents and cancer 6(2):S9, 2011.

Awsthi, A., Mathur, R.K., Saha, B. Immune response to *Leishmania* infection. Indian J. Med. Res. June 2004 pp 238-258.

AZEVEDO, S. K. S.; SILVA, I. M. Plantas medicinais e de uso religioso comercializadas em mercados e fairs livres no Rio de Janeiro, RJ, Brasil. *Acta botânica brasilica*, v. 20, n. 1, p. 185-194, 2006.

BARBOZA, D. C. P. M.; GOMES NETO, C. M. B.; LEAL, D. C.; BITTENCOURT, D. V. V.; CARNEIRO, A. J. B.; SOUZA, B. M. P. S.; OLIVEIRA, L. S.; JULIÂO, F. S.; SOUZA, V. M. M.; FRANKE, C. R. Cohort study in areas at risk of canine visceral leishmaniasis in municipalities in the Metropolitan Region of Salvador, Bahia, Brazil. Revista Brasileira de Saùde Produçao Aninal, v.7, p.152-163, 2006.

BASANO, S.A.;. CAMARGO, L.M.A. American Tegumentary Leishmaniasis: history, epidemiology and control perspectives. Revista Brasileira de Epidemiologia, v.7, p. 328-337, 2004.

Baskar, R., Rajeswari, V., Kumar, T.A. *In vitro* antioxidant studies in leaves of *Annona* species. Indian Journal of experimental biology 45:480-485, 2007

BERGMANN, B.R., COSTA, S.S, MORAES, V.L.G. Brazilian medicinal plants: A rich source of immunomodulatory substances. Brazilian Journal Association for the Advancement of Science, v. 49, p 395-402, 1997.

Bermejo A, Figadere B, Zafra-Polo MC, Barrachina I, Estornell E, Cortes D 2005. Acetogenins from Annonaceae: recent progress in isolation, synthesis and mechanisms of action. *Nat Prod Rep* 22: 269-303.

BHAKUNI, D.S., TEWARI, S., DHAR, M.M. Alkaloids from leaves of *Annona squamosa*. Phytochemistry, v. 11, p. 1819-1822, 1972.

BHAKUNI, D.S., TEWARI, S., DHAR, M.M. Aporphine alkaloids of *Annona squamosa*. Phytochemistry, v. 18, n. 9, p. 1584-1586, 1979.

Blum, J., Desjeux, P., Schwartz, E., Beck, B., Hatz, C. Treatment of cutaneous leishmaniasis among travelers. Journal of antimicrobial chemotherapy 53:158-166, 2004.

BOTELHO, M.A; BASTOS, G.M; FONSECA, S.G.C; MATOS, F.J.A; MONTENEGRO, D; RAO, V.S; BRITO, G.A.C; Antimicrobial activity of the essential oil from *Lippia sidoides*, carvacrol and thymol against oral pathogens. Braz. J Med. Bio. Res., v.40, p. 349-356, 2007.

Boyom, F.F., Fokou, P.V.T., Yamthe, L.R.T., Mfopa, A.N., Kemgne, E.M., Mbacham, W.F., Tsamo, E., Zollo, P.H.A., Gut, J., Rosenthal, P.J. Potent antiplasmodial extracts from Cameroonian Annonaceae. Journal of Ethnopharmacology 134:717-724, 2011.

BRAGA F.G., BOUZADA, M. L. M., FABRI, R. L., MATOS, M. O., MOREIRA, F. O., SCIO, E., COIMBRA, E. S. Antileishmanial and antifungal activity of plants used in traditional medicine in Brazil. Journal of Ethnopharmacology, v. 111, p. 396-402, 2007. Brunton, L.L., Lazo, J.S., Parker, K.L. The pharmacological bases of therapeutics. 11th ed. Rio de Janeiro-RJ, 2006.

CABREIRA, M. A.; PAULA, A. A.; CAMACHO, L.; MARZOCHI, M. C.; XAVIER, S. C.; DA SILVA, A. V. M.; JANSEN, A. M. Canine visceral leishmaniasis in Barra de Guaratiba, Rio de Janeiro, Brazil: assessment of risk factors. Revista do Instituto de Medicina Tropical, v.45, p.79-83,

2003.

Calderon LA, Silva-Jardim I, Zuliani JP, Silva AA, Ciancaglini P, Silva HP, Stàbeli RG. Amazonian Biodiversity: A view of drug Development for leishmaniasis and Malaria. *J Braz Chem Soc* 20: 1011-1023, 2009.

CHAN-BACAB, M. J.; PENA-RODRiGUEZ, L. M. Plant natural products with leishmanial activity. The Royal Society of Chemistry, v. 18, p. 674-688, 2001.

CRAVEIRO, A.C; FERNANDES, A.G; ANDRADE, C.H.S; MATOS, F.J.A; ALENCAR, J.W; MACHADO, M.I.L. Óleos essenciais de plantas do nordeste. Fortaleza, CE: Ediçoes UFC, 1981.

CROFT, S.L; COOMBS, G.H; Leishmaniasis - current chemotherapy and recent advancing the search for novel drugs. Trends in Parasitology, v. 19, n. 11, p. 502-508, 2003.

CROFT, S.L; COOMBS, G.H; Leishmaniasis - current chemotherapy and recent advancing the search for novel drugs. **Trends in Parasitology**, v. 19, n. 11, p. 502-508, 2003.

Dash, G.K., Ganapaty, S., Suresh, P., Panda, S.K., Sahu, S.K. Analgesic and anti-inflammatory activity of *A. squamosal* leaves Indian J at 17(2):32-36, 2001.

DEANE, M.P., DEANE, L.M., Experimental infection of phlebotomus longipalpis in a human case of visceral leishmaniasis.O Hospital, v.46, p.487-489, 1954a

DEANE, M.P., DEANE, L.M., Urban visceral leishmaniasis (the dog and man) in Sobral, Cearà. O Hospital, v.47, p. 75-87, 1955

DEANE, M.P., DEANE, L.M., Observaçoes sobre a transmissào da leishmaniose visceral no cearà. O Hospital, v.48, p.347-364, 1954b

DIETZE, R.; BARROS, G. B.; TEXEIRA, L.; HARRIS, J.; MICHELSON, K.; FALQUETO, A.; COREY, R. Effect of eliminating seropositive canines on the transmission of visceral leishmaniasis in Brazil. Clinical Infectious Disease, v.25, p.1240-1242, 1997.

Dorlo, T.P.C., Balasegaram, M., Beijnen, J.H., Vries, P.J. Miltefosine: a review of its pharmacology and therapeutic efficacy in the treatment of leishmaniasis. Journal of antimicrobial chemotherapy 2012.

ESCOBAR, R.G; Eugenol: Pharmacological and toxicological properties. Advantages and disadvantages of its use. Review Cubana Estomatology, v.39, 2002.

FAGUNDES; F.A; OLIVEIRA; L.B. de; CUNHA; L.C; VALADARES; M.C; *Annona coriacea* induces genotoxic effect in mice. Revista Eletrônica de Farmàcia, v.2, p.24-29, 2005.

Falcao, M.J.C. Contribuicao ao conhecimento quimico de plantas do nordeste *Platymiscium floribundum* VOG. (*Leguminosae*). Defense thesis for a doctorate in Chemistry. Federal University of Ceará, 2003.

Falcao, M.J.C., Pouliquem, Y.B.M., Lima, M.A.S., Gramosa, N.V., Costa-Lotufo, L.V., Militao, G.C.G., Pessoa, C., Moraes, M.O., Silveira, E.R. Cytotoxic flavonoids from *Platymiscium floribundum*. J. Nat Prod. 68:423-426, 2005.

FISA, R.; GALLEGO, M.; CASTILLEJO, S.; AISA, M. J.; SERRA, T.; RIERA, C.; CARRIÓ, J.; GALLEGO, J.; PORTÙS, M. Epidemiology of canine leishmaniosis in Catalonia (Spain): The example of the Priorat focus. Veterinary Parasitology, v.83, p.87-97, 1999.

FRANCA-SILVA, J. C.; DA COSTA, R. T.; SIQUEIRA, A. M.; HADO-COELHO, G. L.; DA COSTA, C. A.; MAYRINK, W.; VIEIRA, E. P.; COSTA, J. S.; GENARO, O.; NASCIMENTO, E. Epidemiology of canine visceral leishmaniasis in the endemic area of Montes Claros Municipality, Minas Gerais State, Brazil. Veterinary Parasitology, v.111, p.161-173, 2003.

Freitas-Junior, L.H., Chatelain, E., Kim, H.A., Siqueira-Neto, J.L. Visceral Leishmaniasis treatment: What do we have, what to we need and how to deliver ir? International journal for parasitology: drugs and drug resistance 2:11-19, 2012.

FUMAGALI, E; GONÇALVES, R. A. C.; MACHADO, M. F. P. S.; VIDOTI, G. J.; OLIVEIRA, A. J. B. Production of secondary metabolites in plant cell and tissue culture: The example of the *Tabernaemontana* and *Aspidosperma* genera. *Revista Brasileira de Farmacognosia*, v. 18, n. 4, p. 627-641, 2008.

FUNASA. National Health Foundation, Ministry of Health. Visceral leishmaniasis in Brazil: current situation, main epidemiological and clinical aspects and control measures. N°06, 2002

George, V.C., Kumar, D.R.N., Raijkumar, V., Suresh, P.K., Kumar, R.A. Quatitative assessment of the relative antineoplastic potential of the n-butanolic leaf extract of *Annona muricata* Linn. in normal and immortalized human cell lines. Asian Pacific J Cancer Prev 13:699-704, 2012

GILL, L.H.S.; BASANO, S.A.; SOUZA, A.A.; SILVA, M.G.S.; BARATA, I.; ISHIKAWA, E.A.; CAMARGO, L.M.A.; Recent observations on the sandfly (Diptera: Psychodidae) fauna of the sate of Rondônia, Western Amazônica, Brazil: the importance of *Psychodopygus davisi* as a vector of zoonotic cutaneus leishmaniasis. Memórias do Instituto Oswaldo Cruz, v.98, p. 751-75, 2003.

GILLESPIE, S., PEARSON R. D., Principles and practice of clinical parasitology. 1st Edition, Copyright, 2001.

GLEYE, C., LAURENS, A., HOCQUEILLER, R., LEPRÉVOTE, O., SERANI, L., CAVÉ, A., Cohibins A and B, acetogenins from roots of *Annona muricata*. Phytochemistry, v. 44, n. 8 p. 1541-1545, 1997.

GLEYE, C., RAYNAUD, S., HOCQUEMILLER, R., LAURENS, A., FOURNEAU, C., SERANI, L., LEPRÉVOTE, O., ROBLOT, F., LEBOEUF, M., FOURNET, A., ARIAS, A.R., FIGADÈRE, B., CAVÉ,A. Muricadienin, muridienins and chatenaytrienins, the early precusors of annonaceous acetogenins. Phytochemistry, v. 47, n. 5, p. 749-754, 1998.

GOBBO-NETO, L.; LOPES, N. P. Medicinal plants: factors influencing the content of secondary metabolites. *QuimicaNova, v.* 30, n. 2, p. 374-381, 2007.

GONTIJO, C.M.F.; MELO, M.N. Visceral leishmaniasis in Brazil: current situation, challenges and perspectives. Revista Brasileira de Epidemiologia, v.7, p. 338-949, 2004.

GRANDIC, S.R., FOURNEAU, C., LAURENS, A., BORIES, C., HOCQUEMILLER, R., LOISEAU, P.M. In vitro antileishmanial activity of acetogenins from Annonaceae. Biomedicine & Pharmacology, v. 58, p. 388-392, 2004.

Grzybowski, A., Tiboni, M., Silva, M.A.N., Chitolina, R.F., Passos, M., Fontana, J.D. The combined action of phytolarvicides for the control of dengue fever vector, *Aedes aegypti*. Revista brasileira de farmacognosia 22:549-557, 2012.

Hamizah, S., Roslida, A.H., Fezah, O., Tan, K.L., Tor, Y.S., Tan, C.I. Chemopreventive potential of *Annona muricata* L Leaves on Chemically-Induced skin papillomagenesis in mice. Asian Pacific Journal of Cancer Prevention 13:2533-2539, 2012.

HOPP, D.C., ALALI, F.Q., GU, Z., McLAUGHLIN, J.L. Mono-THF ring annonaceous acetogenins from *Annona squamosa*. Phytochemistry, v. 47, n. 5, p. 803-809, 1998. *in vitro*. Planta Medica, v. 59, n. 5, p. 474, 1993.

Jaramillo, M.C., Arango, G.J., Gonzàlez, M.C., Robledo, S.M., Velez, I.D. Cytotoxicity and antileishmanial activity of *Annona muricata* pericarp. Fitoterapia 71:183-186, 2000.

Kaleem, M., Asif, M., Ahmed, Q.U., Bano, B. Antidiabetic and antioxidant activity of Annona squamosa extract in streptozotocin-induced diabetic rats. Singapore Med J. 47(8):670-675, 2006.

KAPIL, A. Piperine: A potent inhibitor of *Leishmania donovani* promastigotes

KIM, G., ZENG, L., ALALI, F., ROGERS L.L., WU, F., SASTRODIHARDJO, S., McLAUGHLIN, J.L. Muricoreacin and murihexocin C, mono-tetrahydrofuran acetogenins, from the leaves of *Annona muricata*. Phytochemistry, v. 49, n. 2, p. 565571, 1998.

KONNO, H., OKUNO, Y., MAKABE, H., NOSAKA, K., ONISHI, A., ABE, Y., SUGIMOTO, A., AKAJI, K. Total synthesis of *cis-solamin* A, a mono-tetrahydrifuran acetogenin isolated from *Annona muricata*. Tetrahedron Letters, v. 49, n. 5, p. 782-785, 2008.

KORDALI, S; CAKIR, A; OZER, H; CAKMAKCI, R; KESDEK, M; METE, E. Antifungal, phytotoxic and insecticidal properties of essential oil isolated from *Turkish Origanum acutidens* and its three components, carvacrol, thymol and ρ-cymene. Bioresouce Technology, n. 99, v. 18, p. 8789-8795, 2008

Kumar, A.J., Rekha, T., Devi, S.S., Khannan, M., Jaswanth, A., Gopal, V. Insecticidal activity of ethanolic extract of *Annona squamosal*. Journal of chemical and pharmaceutical research 2(5): 177-180, 2010.

Lima, M.R.F., Luna, J.S., Santos, A.F., Andrade, M.C.C., Sant'Ana, A.E.G., Genet, J., Marquez, B., Neuville, L., Moreau, N. Anti-bacterial activity of some Brazilian medicinal plants. Journal of Ethnopharmacology 105:137-147, 2006.

Luna, J.S., Santos, A.F., Lima, M.R.F., Omena, M.C., Mendonça, F.A.C., Bieber, L.W., Sant'Ana, A.E.G. A study of the larvicidal and molluscicidal activities od some medicinal plants from northeast Brazil. Journal of Ethnopharmacology 97:199-206, 2005.

MAHIOU V, ROBLOT F, HOCQUEMILLER R, CAVE A, ROJAS DE ARIAS A, INCHAUSTI A, YALUFF G, FOURNET A. Aporphine alkaloids from Guatteria foliosa. J Nat Prod, v. 57, p. 890-895, 1994

MARKOWITZ, K., MOYNIHAN, M., LIU, M., KIM, S. Biologic properties of eugenol and zinc oxide-eugenol. Oral Surg Oral Med Oral Pathol, v.73, p. 729-737, 1992.

MARZOCHI, M. C. A., COUTINHO, S. G., SOUZA, W. J., AMENDOEIRA,M.R. Visceral Leishmaniasis (Calazar). Jornal Brasileiro de Medicina. v. 1, n.5, p. 61-84, 1981.

MARZOCHI, M. C. A., Canine visceral leishmaniasis in Rio de Janeiro - Brazil. Cadernos de Saùde Pùblica, v.1, p.432-446, 1985

Mayrink, W., Botelho, A.C.C., Magalhaes, P.A., Batista, S.M., Lima, A.O., Genaro, O., Costa, C.A., Melo, M.N., Michalick, M.S.M., Williams, P., Dias, M., Caiaffa, W.T., Nascimento, E., Machado-Coelho, G.L.L. Immunotherapy, immunochemotherapy and chemotherapy for American cutaneous leishmaniasis treatment. Revista da Sociedade Brasileira de Medicina Tropical 39(1):14-21, Jan-Feb, 2006

Militao, G.C.G., Dantas, I.N.F., Pessoa, C., Falcao, M.J.C., Silveira, E.R., Lima, M.A., Curi, R., Lima, T., Moraes, M.O., Costa-Lotufo, L.V. Induction of apoptosis by pterocarpans from *Platymiscium floribundum* in HL-60 human leukemia cells. Life sciences 78:2409-2417, 2006.

MILTERSTEINER A., MILTERSTEINER D., PEREIRA FILHO N., FROTA A.R., ELY P.B., ZETTLER C.G., MARRONI C.A., MARRONI N.P. Long-term use of quercetin in cirrhotic rats. Acta Cirûrgica Brasileira, n° 8, v. 3, 2003.

MISHRA B. B., KALE R. R., SINGH R. K., TIWARI V. K.. Alkaloids: Future prospective to combat leishmaniasis. Fitoterapia, n° 80, p. 81-90, 2009.

MORAIS, S. M.; BRAZ-FILHO, R. Produtos naturais: estudos quimicos e biológicos. Fortaleza: Ed. UECE, 2007.

MOREIRA JR, E. D.; SOUZA, V. M. M.; SREENIVASAN, M.; LOPES, N.L.; BARRETO, R. B.; CARVALHO, L. P. Peridomestic risk factors for canine leishmaniasis in urban dwellings: new findings from a prospective study in Brazil. American Journal of Tropical Medicine Hygiene, v.69, p.393- 397, 2003.

Motta, J.O.C., Sampaio, R.N.R. A pilot study comparing low-dose liposomal amphotericin B with N-methyl glucamine for the treatment of American cutaneous leishmaniasis. Journal of the European Academy of Dermatology and Venereology 26:331-335, 2012.

Mrita, S., Singh, D.K. Molluscicidal activity of the custard apple (Annona squamosa L.) alone and in combination with other plant derived molluscicides. Journal of herbs, spices & medicinal plants 8 (1): 23-29, 2001.

Mujeeb, M., Alam, K.S., Mohd, A., Abhishek, M., Aftab, A. Antidiabetic activity of the aqueous extract of *Annona squamosa* in streptozotocin induced hyperglycemic rats. The pharma research 2:59-63, 2009.

MUZITANO, M.F., TINOCO, L.W., GUETTE, C., KAISER, C.R., ROSSI- BERGMANN, B., COSTA, S.S. The altileishmanicidal of usual flavonoids from *Kalanchoe pinnata*. Phytochemistry, n. 67, p. 2071-2077, 2006.

NUNES V.L.B., GALATI E.A.B., NUNES D.B., ZINEZZI R.O., SAVANI E.S.M.M., ISHIKAWA E., CAMARGO M.C.G.O., D'AURIA S.R.N., CRISTALDO G. & ROCHA H.C. Occurrence of canine visceral leishmaniasis in an agricultural settlement in the state of Mato Grosso do Sul, Brazil. **Revista da Sociedade Brasileira de Medicina Tropical,** v.34, p.301-302, 2001.

Nunes, C.M., Pires, M.M., Silva, K.M., Assis, F.D., Gonçalves-Filho, J., Perri, S.H. Relationship between dog culling and incidence of human visceral leishmaniasis in an edemic area. Veterinary Parasitology 28:131-133, 2010.

Nwokocha, C.R., Owu, D.U., Gordon, A., Thaxter, K., McCalla, G., Ozolua, R.I., Young, L. Possible mechanisms of action of the hypotensive effect of *Annona muricata* (soursop) in normotensive Sprague-Dawley rats. Pharmaceutical Biology *In print.*

OLIVEIRA, C.D.L., ASSUNÇÂO, R.M., REIS, I.A., PROIETTI, F.A., Spatial distribution of human and canine visceral leishmaniasis in Belo Horizonte, Minas Gerais

Gerais State, Brazil, 1994-1997. **Cad. Saùde Pùblica, Rio de Janeiro**, v.17, n.5, p.1231-1239, 2001

OLIVEIRA-FREITAS, E., CASAS, C.P., BORJA-CABRERA, G.P., SANTOS, F.N., NICO, D., SOUZA, L.O.P., TINOCO, L.W., SILVA, B.P., PALATNIK, M., PARENTE, J.P., PALATNIK-DE-SOUSA, C.B. Acylated and deacylated *saponins* of *Quillaja saponaria* mixture as adjuvants for the FML-vaccine visceral leishmaniasis. Vaccine, n. 24, p. 3909-3920, 2006.

Padma, P., Pramod, N.P., Thyagarajan, S.P., Khosa, R.L. Effect of the extract of *Annona muricata* and *Petunia nyctaginiflora* on Herpes simplex virus. Journal of Ethnopharmacology 61:81-83, 1998.

Paladin Labs Inc. Application for inclusion of Miltefosine on WHO model list of essential medicines. 2010. http://www.who.int/selection medicines/committees/expert/18/applications/Miltefosine application.pdf

Pandley, N., Barve, D. Phytochemical and pharmacological review of *Annona squamosa* Linn. International Journal of research in pharmaceutical and biomedical science. 2:1404-1412, 2011.

PARANHOS-SILVA, M.; NASCIMENTO, E. G.; MELRO, M. C. B. F.; OLIVEIRA, G. C. S.; DOS SANTOS, W. L. C.; PONTES-DECARVALHO, L. C.; OLIVEIRA- DOS-SANTOS, A. J. Cohort study on canine emigration and Leishmania infection in an endemic area for visceral leishmaniasis. Implications for disease control. Acta Tropica, v.69, p.75-83, 1998.

Patel, R., Jain, S., Malviya, S., Ahmed, A. Pharmacological review of leaves of "*Annona squamosal*" in G.I. tract ulcer I albino wistar rats. World Journal of pharmacy and pharmaceutical sciences 2:499-524, 2012.

PATHAK, D., PATHAK, K., SINGLA, A.K. Flavonoids as medicinal agents: recent advances. Fitoterapia, v. 57, n. 5, p. 371-389, 1991.

Paula, C.D.R., Sampaio, J.H.D., Cardozo, D.R., Sampaio, R.N.R. Comparative study of the efficacy of pentamidine isethionate administered in three doses over one week and N-methyl-glucamine 20mgSbV/kg/day for 20 days for the treatment of the cutaneous form of American tegumentary leishmaniasis. Revista da sociedade brasileira de medicina Tropical 36(3): 365-371.

PENNA, H.A. Visceral leishmaniasis in Brazil. Brasil Médico, v.18, p.940-950, 1934 PHILLIPSON, J.D., WRIGHT, C.W. Medicinal plants against protozoal diseases. Trans. Roy. Soc. Trop. Med. Hyg,. v. 85, p. 18-21, 1991.

PIAZZA, R.M.F; ANDRADE, H.F; UMEZAWA, E.S; KATZIN, M; STOLF, A.M.S. *In situ* immunoassay for the assessment of *Trypanosoma cruzi* interiorization and growth in cultured cells. Acta Trop. 57, 301-306, 1994

QUEIROZ EF, ROBLOT F, CAVE A, PAULO MD, FOURNET A . Pessoine and spinosine, two catecholic berbines from Annona spinescens. J Nat Prod, v.59, p.438440, 1996

RAB, M. A.; FRAME, I. A.; EVANS, D. A. The role of dogs in the epidemiology of human visceral leishmaniasis in northern Parkistan. Transactions of the Royal Society of Tropical Medicine and Hygiene, v.89, p.612-615, 1995.

RATH, S., TRIVELIN, L.A., IMBRUNITO, T.R., TOMAZELA, D.M., JESÙS, M.N., MARZAL, P.C. Antimonials Used in the Treatment of Leishmaniasis: State of the Art. **Quimica Nova**, v. 26, n. 4, p. 550-555, 2003.

ROBLEDO, S., OSORIO, E., MUNOZ, D., JARAMILLO, L.M., RESTREPO, A., ARANGO, G. In Vitro and In Vivo Cytotoxicities and Antileishmanial Activities of Thymol and Hemisynthetic Derivatives. Antimicrob Agents Chemother. V.49, n. 4, p. 1652-1655, 2005.

ROCHA, L.G.; ALMEIDA, J.R.G.S; MACÊDO, R.O; BARBOSA-FILHO, J.M; A review of natural products with antileishmanial activity. Phytomedicine, v.12, p. 514535, 2005.

Rondon FC, Bevilaqua CM, Franke CR, Barros RS, Oliveira FR, Alcântara AC, Diniz AT. Cross-sectional serological study of canine Leishmania infection in Fortaleza, Cearâ state, Brazil. Vet Parasitol. 2008155(1-2):24-31.

SESSA, P. A., FALQUETO, A., VAREJAO, J.B.M., Attempt to control American tegumentary leishmaniasis by treating sick dogs. Cad. Saùde Pùblica, v. 10, n. 4, p. 457-463, 1994.

SIMÔES, C. M. O.; SCHENKEL, E. P.; GOSMANN, G.; MELLO, J. C. P.; MENTZ, L. A.; PETROVICK, P.R. Farmacognosia: da planta ao medicamento. 5 ed. Porto Alegre/Florianópolis: Editora da Universidade UFRGS / Editora da UFSC, 2004.

Soto, J., Arana, B.A., Toledo, J., Rizzo, N., Veja, J.C., Diaz, A., Luz, M., Gutierres, P., Arboleda, M., Berman, J.D., Junge, K., Engel, J., Sindermann, H. Miltefosine for new word cutaneous leishmaniasis. Clinical Infectious diseases 38:1266-1272, 2004.

Souza MMC, Bevilaqua CML, Morais SM, Costa CTC, Silva ARA, Braz-Filho R. Anthelmintic acetogenin from *Annona squamosa* L. seeds. An Acad Bras Cien 80:271277, 2007.

Sundar, S., Singh, A., Rai, M., Prajapati, V.K., Singh, A.K., Ostyn, B., Boelaert, M., Dujardin, J., Chakravarty, J. Efficacy of Miltefosine in the treatment of visceral leishmaniasis after a decade of use in India. Clinical diseases advance. Accepted Manuscript, 2012.

TASWELL, C. Limiting dilution assays for the determination of immunocompetent cell frequencies III. Validity tests for the single-hit Poisson model. J. Immunol. Meth., 72: 29-40, 1984.

Tempone, A.G., Andrade Jr, H.F. Nanoformulations of pentavalent antimony entrapped in phosphatidylserine-liposomes demonstrate highest efficacy against experimental visceral leishmaniasis. Rev. Inst. Adolfo Lutz 67(2):131-136, 2008.

TEMPONE, A.G; BORBOREMA, S.E.T; ANDRADE Jr, H.F.de; GUALDA; N.C.de A; YOGI; A; CRAVALHO; C.S; BACHIEGA; D; LUPO; F.N; BONOTTO; S.V; FISCHER; D.C.H. Antiprotozoal activity of Brazilian plant extracts from isoquinoline alkaloids-producing families. Phytomedicine, v.12, p. 382-390, 2005.

TITUS, R.G., CEREDIG, R., CEROTTINI, J.C., LOUIS, J.A. Therapeutic effect of anti-L3T4 monoclonal antibody GK 1.5 on cutaneous leishmaniasis in genetically- susceptible BALB/c mice. J. Immunol., 135: 2108-2114, 1985.

Torres, M.P., Rachagani, S., Purohit, V., Pandey, P., Joshi, S., Moore, E.D., Johansson, S.L., Singh, P.K., Ganti, A.K., Batra, S.K. Graviola: A novel promising natural-derived drug that inhibits tumorigenicity and metastasis of pancreatic cancer cells *in vitro* and *in vivo* through altering cell metabolism. Cancer letters 323:29-40, 2012.

UEDA-NAKAMURA, T; MENDONÇA-FILHO, R.R; MORGADO-DiAZ, J.A; MAZA, P.K; DIAS, B.P; CORTEZ, D.A.G; ALVIANO, D.S; ROSA, M.S.S; LOPES, A.H.C.S; ALVIANO, C.S; NAKAMURA, C.V. Antileishmanial activity of Eugenol- rich essential oil from *Ocimum gratissimum*. Parasitology Internetional, n. 55, p. 99105, 2006.

Upadhyay, R.K., Ahmad, S. Ethno-medicinal plants and their pharmaceutical potential. Journal of pharmacy research. 5(4):2162-2173, 2012.

Valillo, M.I., Caruso, M.F.S., Takemoto, E., Pimentel, S. Chemical and physico-chemical characterization of the oil from the seeds of *Platymiscium floribundum* Vog. (Sacambu), harvested at the stage of development and at the time of physiological maturation. Rev. Inst. Flor. 19(2):73-80, 2007.

Van Griensven, J., Diro, E. Visceral Leishmaniasis. Infect Dis Clin N Am 26:309-322, 2012.

VEIGA JÛNIOR, V. F; PINTO A.C; MACIEL. A. M. Medicinal plants: Safe cures? Quimica Nova, v. 28, n. 3, p. 519-528, 2005

VOULDOUKIS, I., ROUGIER, S., DUGAS, B., PINO, P., MAZIER, D., WOEHRLÉ, F. Canine visceral leishmaniasis: Comparison of in vitro leishmanicidal activity of marbofloxacin meglumine antimoniate and sodium stibogluconate.Veterinary Parasitology, v. 135, p. 137-146, 2006

WAECHTER, A., YALUFF, G., INCHAUSTI, A., ARIAS, A.R., HOCQUEMILLER, R., CAVÉ, A., FOURNET, A. Leishmanicidal and trypanocidal activities of acetogenins isolated from *Annona glauca*. Phytotherapy Research, v. 12, p. 541-544, 1998.

WORLD HEALTH ORGANIZATION (WHO).

http://www.who.int/zoonoses/diseases/leishmaniasis/en/, accessed August 2008

WU, B.N; HWANG, T.L; LIAO, C.F; CHEN, M.I.J. Vaninolol: a newselective bête B- adrenergic antagonist derived from vanillin. Biochemical Pharmacology, v.48, p. 101109, 1994.

Srivastava, S., Lal, V.K., Pant, K.K. Medicinal potential of *Annona squamosa*: At a glance. Journal of pharmacy research 4:4596-4598, 2011.

YU, J., GUI, H., LUO, X., SUN, L. Murihexol, a linear acetogenin from *Annona muricata*. Phytochemistry, v. 49, n. 6, p. 1689-1692, 1998.

Yuan, S.S., Chang, H.L., Chen, H.W., Yeh, T., Kao, Y., Lin, K., Wu, Y., Su, J.

Annonacin, a mono tetrahydrofuran acetogenin, arrests cancer cells at the G1 phase and causes cytotoxicity in a Baxand caspase-3-related pathway. Life sciences, 72:28532861, 2003

Kishore, N., Mishra, B.B., Tripathi, V., Tiwari, V.K. Alkaloids as potential anti- tubercular agents. Phytotherapy 80:149-163, 2009.

Min, H., Chung, H., Kim, E., Kim, S., Park, E., Lee, S.k. Inhibition of cell growth and potential of tumor necrosis factor-α (TNF-α)-induced apoptosis by phenanthroindolizidine alkaloid anthophine in human colon cancer cells. Biochemical Pharmacology 80:1356-1364, 2010.

Satou, T., Koga, M., Matsuhashi, R., Koike, K., Tada, I., Nikaido, T. Assay of nematocidal activity of isoquinoline alkaloids using third-stage lavae *of Strongyloides ratti* and *S. venezuelensis*. Veterinary Parasitology 104:131-138, 2003.

Bagalwa, J.M., Voutquenne-Nazabadioko, L., Sayagh, C., Bashwira, A.S. Evaluation of the biological activity of the molluscicidal fraction of *Solanum sisymbriifolium* against non target organisms. Fitoterapia 81:767-771, 2010.

Maneerat, W., Phakhodee, W., Ritthiwigrom, T., Cheenpracha, S., Promgool, T., Yossathera, K., Deachathai, S., Laphookhieo, S. Antibacterial carbazole alkaloids from *Clausena harmandiana* twigs. Fitoterapia 83:1110-1114, 2012.

Manhas, M.S., Ganguly, S.N., Mukherjee, S., Jain, A.K., Bose, A.K. Microwave initiated reactions: Pechmann coumarin synthesis Biginelli reaction, and acylation. Tetrahedron Letters 47:2423-2425, 2005.

Hoult, J.R.S., Payat, M. Pharmacological and biochemical actions of simple coumarins: Natural products with therapeutic potential. General Pharmacology: The vascular system 27:713-722, 1996.

Kontogiorgis, C., Detsi, A., Hadjipavlou-Litina, D. Coumarin-based drugs: a patent review (2008-present). Expert opinion on therapeutic patents 22:437-454, 22012.

Kim, N.H., Kim, S., Oh, J.S., Lee, S., Kim, Y.K. Anti-mitotic potential of 7- diethylamino-3(2'-benzoxazolyl)-coumarin in 5-fluorouracil-resistant human gastric cancer cell line SNU620/5-FU. Biochemical and Biophysical research communications 418:616-621, 2012.

Huang, L., Yuan, X., Yu, D., Lee, K.H., Chen, C.H. Mechanism of action and resistant profile of anti-HIV-1 coumarin derivatives. Virology 332:623-628, 2005.

Jaiswal, S., Bhattacharya, K., Sullivan, M., Walsh, M., Creaven, B., Laffir, F., Duffy, B., McHale, P. Non-cytotoxic antibacterial silver-coumarin complex doped sol-gel coatings. Colloids and surfaces B: Biointerfaces (2010), doi:10.1016/j.colsurfb.2012.07.047

Gilani, A.H., Shaheen, F., Saeed, S.A., Bibi, S., Irfanullah, Sadiq, M., Faizi, S. Hypotensive action of coumarin glycosides from *Daucus carota*. Phytomedicine 7:423426, 2000.

Yang, Y.J., Lee, H.J., Lee, B.K., Lim, S.C., Lee, C.K., Lee, M.K. Effects of scoporone on dopamine release I PC12 cells. Phytotherapy 81:497-502, 2010.

Choi, Y.H., Yan, G.H., Anti-allergic effects of scoporone on mast cell-mediated allergy model. Phytomedicine 16:1089-1094, 2009.

Ferreira, M.E., Arias, A.R.,Yaluff, G., Bilbao, N.V., Nakayama, H., Torres, S., Schinini, A., Guy, I., Heinzen, H., Fournet, A. Antileishmanial activity of furoquinolines and coumarins from *Helietta apiculata*. Phytomedicine 17:375-378, 2010

Napolitano, H.B., Silva, M., Ellena, J., Rodrigues, B.D.G., Almeida, A.L.C., Vieira, P.C., Oliva, G., Thiemann, O.H. Aurapten, a coumarin with growth inhibition against *Leishmania major* promastigotes. Brazilian Journal of Medical and Biological Research 37:1847-1852, 2004.

Choi, W.S., Jang, D.Y., Nam, S.W., Park, B.S., Lee, H., Lee, S.E. Antiulcerogenic activity of scoparone on HCl/Ethanol-induced gastritis in rats. J. Korean Soc Appl Biol Chem 55:159-163, 2012.

Fang, Y., Li, Z., Watanabe, Y. Pharmacokinetics of a novel anti-asthmatic, scoporone, in the rabbit serum assessed by a simple HPLC method. Journal of ethnopharmacology 86:127-130, 2003.

Pires, N.R., Cunha, P.L.R., Paula, R.C.M., Feitosa, J.P.A., Jamacaru, F.V.F., Filho, M.O.M. Ophthalmic viscoelastics: Comparison between commercial ones and formulations of galactomannan from *Dimorphandra gardneria*. Quimica nova 33:1709-1713, 2010.

Cunha, P.L.R., Vieira, I.G.P., Arriaga, A.M.C., Paula, R.C.M., Feitosa, J.P.A. Isolation and characterization of galactomannan from *Dimorphandra gardneriana* Tul. Seeds as a portential guar gum substitute. Food Hydrocolloids 23:880-885, 2009.

Solano-Galego, L., Koutinas, A., Miró, G., Cardoso, L., Pennisi, M.G., Ferrer, L., Bourdeau, P., Oliva, G., Baneth, G. Directions for the diagnosis, clinical staging, treatment and prevention of canine leishmaniasis. Veterinary Parasitology 165:1-18, 2009.

Borska, S., Chmielewska, M., Wysocka, T., Drag-Zalesinka, M., Zabel, M., Dziegiel, P. *In vitro* effect of quercetin on human gastric carcinoma: Targeting cancer cell death and MDR. Food and chemical toxicology 50:3375-3383, 2012.

Lin, C., Leu, Y., Al-Suwayeh, A., Ku, M., Hwang, T., Fang, J. Anti-inflammatory activity and percutaneous absorption of quercetin and its polymethoxylated compound and glycosides: The relationships to chemical structures. European journal of pharmaceutical science, 20120 Article in press.

Savov, V.M., Galabov, A.S., Tantcheva, L.P., Mileva, M.M., Pavlova, E.L., Stoeva, E.S., Braykova, A.A. Effects of rutin and quercetin on monooxygenase activities in experimental influenza virus infection. Experimental and toxicologic pathology 58:5964, 2006.

Sen, N., Das, B.B., Ganguly, A., Banerjee, B., Sen, T., Majumder, H.K. *Leishmania donovani*: Intracellular ATP level regulates apoptosis-like death in luteolin induced dyskinetoplastid cells. Experimental Parasitology 114:204-212, 2006.

Silva, E.R., Maquiaveli, C.C., Magalhaes, P.P. The Ieishmanicidal flavonols quercetin and quercetri target *Leishmania (Leishmania) amazonensis* arginase. Experimental Parasitology 130:183-188, 2012.

Shen, S., Hsu, W., Lee, C., Chang, W., Wu, S. Buckwheat extracts (*Fagopyrum tataricum*) and rutin attenuate Th2 cytokines production and cellular allergic effects in vitro and in vivo. Journal of functional foods 4:793-799, 2012.

Marcarini, J.C., Tsuboy, M.S.F., Luiz, R.C., Ribeiro, L.R., Hoffmann-Campo, C.B., Mantovani, M.S. Investigation of cytotoxic, apoptosis-inducing, genotoxic and protective effects of the flavonoid rutin in HTC hepatic cells. Experimental and toxicology pathology 63:459-465, 2011.

Kim, G., Kwon, Y., Jang, H. Protective mechanism of quercetin and rutin on 2,2'- azobis(2-amidinopropane) dihydrochloride or Cu^{2+} -induced oxidative stress in HepG2 cells. Toxicology in vitro 25:138-144, 2011.

Selloum, L., Bouriche, H., Tigrine, C., Boudoukha, C. Anti-inflammatory effect of rutin on rat paw oedema, and on neutrophils chemotaxis and degranulation. Exp Toxic pathol 54:313-318, 2003.

Nair, V.D., Gopi, R., Mohankumar, M., Kavina, J., Panneerselvam, R. Effect of triadimefon: a triazole fungicide on oxidative stress defense system and eugenol content in *Ocimum tenuiflorum* L. Acta physiol Plant 34:599-605, 2012.

Pessoa, L.M., Morais, S.M., Bevilaqua, C.M.L., Luciano, J.H.S. Anthelmintic activity of essential oil of *Ocimum gratissimum* Linn. And eugenol against *Haemonchus contortus*. Veterinary Parasitology 109:59-63, 2002.

Maciel, M.V., Morais, S.M., Bevilaqua, C.M.L., Silva, R.A., Barros, R.S., Sousa, R.N., Sousa, L.C., Brito, E.S., Souza-Neto, M.A. Chemical composition of *Eucalyptus* spp. Essential oils and their insecticidal effects on *Lutzomyia longipalpis*. Veterinary Parasitology 167:1-7, 2010.

Guarda, A., Rubilar, J.F., Miltz, J., Galotto, M.J. The antimicrobial activity of microencapsulated thymol and carvacrol. Internetional Journal of Food Microbiology 146:144-150, 2011.

Szentandràssy, N., Szigeti, G., Szegedi, C., Sàrkozi, S., Magyar, J., Banyasz, T., Csernoch, L., Kovacs, L., Nanasi, P.P., Jona, I. Effect of thymol on calcium handling in mammalian ventricular myocardium. Life Sciences 74:909-921.

Riella, K.R., Marinho, R.R., Santos, J.S., Pereira-Filho, R.N., Cardoso, J.C., Albuquerque-Junior, R.L.C., Thomazzi, S.M. Anti-inflammatory and cicatrizing activities of thymol, a monoterpene of the essential oil from *Lippia gracilis*, in rodents. Journal of Ethnopharmacology 143:656-663, 2012.

Ahmad, A., Khan, A., Yousuf, S., Khan, L.A., Manzoor, N. Proton translocating ATPase mediated fungicidal activity of eugenol and thymol. Phytotherapy 81:1157-1162, 2010.

Underger, U., Basaran, A., Degen, G.H., Basaran, N. Antioxidant activities of major thyme ingredients and lack of (oxidative) DNA damage in V79 Chinese hamster lung fibroblast cells ar low levels of carvacrol and thymol. Food and chemical toxicology 47:2037-2043, 2009.

Medeiros, M.G.F., Silva, A.C., Citó, A.M.G.L., Borges, A.R., Lima, S.G., Lopes, J.A.D., Figueiredo,

R.C.B.Q. In vitro antileishmanial activity and cytotoxicity of essential oil from *Lippia sidoides* Cham. Parasitology International 60:237-241, 2011.

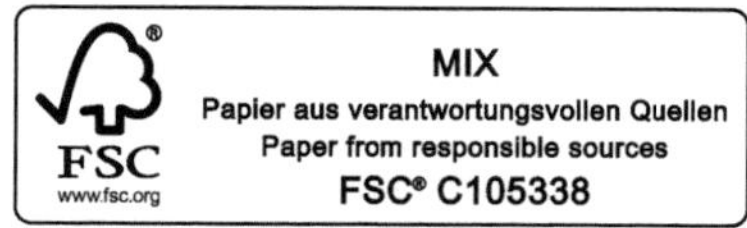

Printed by Books on Demand GmbH, Norderstedt / Germany